Lens Prescribing, and Care of the Keratoconus Patient

Timothy M. Nivala, O.D.

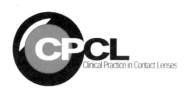

Series Editors

Gerald E. Lowther, O.D., Ph.D.
The Borish Center for Ophthalmic Research,
Indiana School of Optometry, Bloomington

Charles D. Leahy, O.D., M.S.
Assistant Clinical Professor of Optometry,
New England College of Optometry, Boston;
Contact Lens Service, Massachusetts Eye and
Ear Infirmary, Boston

Other titles in the Clinical Practice in Contact Lenses series:

Lowther: *Dryness, Tears, and Contact Lens Wear* (1997)
Begley: *RGP Lens Fitting* (Forthcoming)

Diagnosis, Contact Lens Prescribing, and Care of the Keratoconus Patient

Clinical Practice in Contact Lenses

Karla Zadnik, O.D., Ph.D.
Associate Professor, College of Optometry,
The Ohio State University, Columbus

Joseph T. Barr, O.D., M.S.
Associate Professor, College of Optometry,
The Ohio State University, Columbus

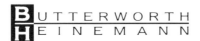

Boston Oxford Auckland Johannesburg Melbourne New Delhi

Every effort has been made to ensure that the drug dosage schedules within this text are accurate and conform to standards accepted at time of publication. However, as treatment recommendations vary in the light of continuing research and clinical experience, the reader is advised to verify drug dosage schedules herein with infor-mation found on product information sheets. This is especially true in cases of new or infrequently used drugs.

 Recognizing the importance of preserving what has been written, Butterworth–Heinemann prints its books on acid-free paper whenever possible.

 Butterworth–Heinemann supports the efforts of American Forests and the Global ReLeaf program in its campaign for the betterment of trees, forests, and our environment.

Library of Congress Cataloging-in-Publication Data
Zadnik, Karla.
   Diagnosis, contact lens prescribing, and care of the keratoconus
   patient / Karla Zadnik, Joseph T. Barr
      p.   cm. — (Clinical practice in contact lenses)
   Includes bibliographical references and index.
   ISBN 0-7506-9676-1
   1. Keratoconus.   2. Contact lenses.   I. Barr, Joseph T.
   II. Title.   III. Series.
   [DNLM: 1. Keratoconus—diagnosis.   2. Keratoconus—therapy.
   3. Contact Lenses.   WW 220 Z17d 1999]
   RE339.Z33   1999
   617.7'19—dc21
   DNLM/DLC
   for Library of Congress   98-50994
                                                                  CIP

British Library Cataloguing-in-Publication Data
A catalogue record for this book is available from the British Library.

The publisher offers special discounts on bulk orders of this book.
For information, please contact:

Manager of Special Sales
Butterworth–Heinemann
225 Wildwood Avenue
Woburn, MA 01801-2041
Tel: 781-904-2500
Fax: 781-904-2620

For information on all B-H medical publications available, contact our
World Wide Web home page at: http://www.bh.com

10 9 8 7 6 5 4 3 2 1

Printed in the United States of America

Contents

Series Preface

This second volume in the Clinical Practice in Contact Lenses series addresses the condition of keratoconus. One of the goals of the series is to make the clinician knowledgeable and comfortable in handling common clinical challenges. Nowhere do the art and science of contact lens practice come together more intimately than in the initial fitting and long-term care of keratoconus patients.

The optometrist is often the only source of treatment and education for keratoconus patients. Even those patients presented with a diagnosis made elsewhere usually cannot remember the name of the condition and have been told little about treatment or prognosis. Educating the patient is a necessary step in the initiation of treatment and a crucial part of its ongoing success. By stressing the scientific aspects of their presentation, Drs. Zadnik and Barr present a comprehensive body of knowledge from which a clinician can educate his or her patients with authority and care for them with confidence. Fitting procedures and modifications are presented with reviews of what is known in the field rather than as anecdotal experience of the authors or others. The authors' involvement in the only prospective, multicenter study on keratoconus, recently extended for five years, promises important contributions to the future care of keratoconus patients.

Gerald E. Lowther

Charles D. Leahy

Preface

This volume of the series on Clinical Practice in Contact Lenses discusses the corneal disease keratoconus. It includes epidemiological information on the disease as well as presenting more conventional information on the fitting of contact lenses and management of contact lens correction in keratoconus.

It is very data-driven; we have concentrated on presenting what we definitely know about keratoconus rather than what we anecdotally believe. There is certainly some information that is derived from clinical observation, but we hope that this volume will stimulate the reader to also consult the relevant published scientific papers on the topic of keratoconus if he or she wants to know even more.

We would like to thank all the members of the CLEK Study Group, especially Tim Edrington and Mae Gordon, for the continuing intellectual stimulation that makes the study of keratoconus so interesting.

Thanks to Janis M. Cotter, O.D., the Executive Vice President of the Boston Foundation for Sight, for the section on gas permeable scleral lenses.

Karla Zadnik

Joseph T. Barr

Diagnosis, Contact Lens Prescribing, and Care of the Keratoconus Patient

Introduction

Keratoconus is a slowly progressive, noninflammatory axial thinning and distortion of the cornea that is usually bilateral but asymmetric.[1] The cause of keratoconus is unknown, but it is classically described as being associated with certain systemic diseases, such as atopy and connective tissue disorders. Typically, somewhere between the teens and thirties, the disease manifests itself initially as irregular astigmatism, which progresses with increasing corneal curvature and corneal scarring. The management of keratoconus includes refractive error correction, first with spectacles and later with contact lenses, and eventually may require penetrating keratoplasty.

Incidence and Prevalence

Estimates of the prevalence of keratoconus vary from 4 to 108 per 100,000 population.[2, 3] Hofstetter's[3] high estimate is based on keratoscopy results alone and probably includes nonkeratoconic cases of high or irregular astigmatism. In a population-based study over a period of 48 years (1935–1982) in Olmsted County, Minnesota, Kennedy and associates[4] found an average annual incidence of 2 per 100,000 and a prevalence rate of 54.5 per 100,000 population. The traditional literature reports higher prevalence in females.[5] More recent investigators report a majority of males in clinic-based keratoconus populations,[6, 7] although these differences are not statistically significant.

Etiology

The etiology of keratoconus has been investigated frequently but is still largely unknown. It has been described in association with a large variety of systemic diseases and other factors. These include some of the connective tissue disorders, primarily Ehlers-Danlos syndrome and osteogenesis imperfecta, but also oculodentodigital syndrome, Rieger's syndrome, Marfan's syndrome, and focal dermal hypoplasia[8] as well as trisomy 21 (Down syndrome),[9] infantile tapetoretinal degeneration (Leber's congenital amaurosis),[10] atopic disease,[11–14] and corneal trauma in the form of hard contact lens wear[15–18] or eye rubbing.[19–21] A recent survey of almost 1,600 keratoconus patients did not reveal important associations between keratoconus and these rare systemic diseases.[7]

Several of the associated factors and systemic diseases either directly or indirectly implicate decreased or abnormal ocular rigidity. Hartstein and Becker[22] appeared to confirm this impression by measuring low scleral rigidity values in a very small number of eyes with keratoconus and comparing them to normal rigid contact lens wearers, and Davies and Ruben[23] and Brooks et al.[24] agreed. Foster and Yamamoto[25] measured ocular rigidity in larger numbers of keratoconus patients without accompanying systemic connective tissue disease and found no statistically significant difference between study groups with mild-to-moderate keratoconus and normal or transplanted corneas, except in eyes with keratoconus exhibiting greater than 60% corneal thinning. Investigation of the biomechanical strength of the cornea with keratoconus revealed that the tensile strength of the cornea is decreased in keratoconus, out of proportion to that predicted by corneal thinning alone.[26]

Although work is ongoing in the investigation of biochemical and pathological changes at the structural and cellular levels of the cornea,[27–31] a specific mechanism for the development of keratoconus and its relationship to heredity or environment has not been forthcoming. It has been found that abnormal enzyme levels are found in keratoconus patients' corneal and conjunctival epithelium compared to that of normals.[32–34]

The links between keratoconus and eye rubbing,[19–21] with estimates of the prevalence of significant eye rubbing ranging from 66% to 73% in keratoconus patients, would blame increased trauma to the anterior segment for the development of keratoconus. Baseline data from the Collaborative Longitudinal Evaluation of Keratoconus (CLEK) Study indicate that of the 1,207 patients who responded to the eye rubbing question, 582 patients (48.2%) reported rubbing both eyes vigorously, while only 27 patients (2.2%) reported rubbing only one eye vigorously. Five hundred fifty-nine patients (46.3%) did not report eye rubbing in either eye. Thirty-nine patients (3.2%) were unsure whether they rub their eyes.[35]

This theory gains credence from the increased prevalence of atopic disease associated with keratoconus,[11–14] which presumably results in increased symptoms of ocular itching, partly alleviated by eye rubbing; however, other workers have not demonstrated a significant association between atopy and keratoconus.[36, 37] Eye rubbing also can be postulated as the cause of keratoconus seen in patients with trisomy 21 (Down syndrome) and infantile tapetoretinal degeneration (Leber's congenital amaurosis); both groups exhibit an incidence of keratoconus far greater than that seen in the general population and, perhaps coincidentally, engage in frequent, vigorous eye rubbing.

The observation of keratoconus in identical twins, however limited, indicates a role for heredity. A total of five sets of identical twins with keratoconus have been reported in the international ophthalmic literature, with one reported case in the United States.[38] The best study on the heredity of keratoconus was conducted by Hammerstein.[39] The subject population of this prospective study included 52 families, each containing one proband with keratoconus. Nineteen percent of the families had more than two members with keratoconus. Given autosomal dominance and complete penetrance, 50% of the siblings would be expected to have keratoconus. This result would indicate approximately 20% penetrance, if autosomal dominance were the mode of transmission.

Recently, studies of 30 family members of five keratoconus patients have shown related corneal abnormalities, such as central steepening, inferior corneal steepening, and anisometropia, perhaps indicating the variable expression of the keratoconus phenotype.[40]

Symptomatology

The typical patient with undiagnosed keratoconus complains of deteriorating vision, usually in one eye first, both at distance and near. Near visual acuity may improve if the patient squints or holds printed material closer. Keratoconus patients often report monocular diplopia, multiple images, or ghosting of images and often relate a history of frequent refractive correction changes without much improvement in visual acuity. Patients may also report irritative symptoms, such as intolerance of glare, photophobia, and recurrent foreign body sensation.

Even with appropriate contact lens correction, keratoconus patients often report fluctuating vision throughout the day and day to day, although the measurement of visual acuity in keratoconus patients is highly repeatable.[41] In addition, keratoconus patients who wear rigid contact lenses are typically very dependent on their lenses and can become quite frustrated during periods when the lenses are not comfortable or contact lens wearing time is reduced.

Early Signs

Keratoconus usually is bilateral. Estimates of the prevalence of unilateral keratoconus are not reliable because of the asymmetric nature of the disease. Many unilateral cases go on to develop disease in the second eye. Kennedy and associates,[4] for example, report initial unilateral disease at the time of diagnosis in 26 of 61 patients (41%), and 6 of these 26 patients (23%) went on to develop keratoconus in the unaffected eye during the 48-year period of follow-up. Our recent survey reported that 13% of the patients previously diagnosed with keratoconus or diagnosed with keratoconus at the survey visit were reported to have unilateral corneal irregularity at the time of examination as evidenced by irregular keratometric mires, an irregular retinoscopic reflex, and/or an irregular ophthalmoscopic red reflex. Fifty-one percent of the unilateral cases had been diagnosed more than 5 years prior to the date of their examination, indicating that if corneal irregularity develops in the fellow eye, it may occur after a substantial interval of time; however, we did not require assessment of the fellow eye by more sophisticated topographic techniques.

Vision typically improves over the uncorrected or spectacle-corrected level with pinhole or stenopaic slit testing but does not improve adequately with a change in spectacle refraction. Routine contrast sensitivity testing may reveal abnormalities, even before visual acuity decreases.[42–45] Refractive examination reveals moderate, irregular myopic, or mixed astigmatism, if, indeed, refraction with meaningful results is even possible. A scissoring reflex is often noted on retinoscopy.[46]

Slit Lamp Biomicroscopic Signs

Several characteristic features can be seen on biomicroscopy. These include an inferiorly displaced,[47] thinned protrusion of the cornea, visually evident corneal thinning over the apex (Plate 1), Vogt's[48] striae at the level of Descemet's membrane (Plate 2), superficial scars at the level of Bowman's membrane (see Plate 1), and Fleischer's ring (of iron), either full or partial (Plate 3). Vogt's striae can be thought of as stretch marks in the posterior cornea, that form as the cornea protrudes. They are usually vertical but are described as being parallel to the meridian of greatest curvature. Vogt's striae may disappear with transient pressure applied to the globe through the upper lid and may be more easily seen through a rigid gas permeable lens.

Most studies do not report on the prevalence of these slit lamp signs in keratoconus. We have found that a majority of keratoconic eyes may not show individual pathognomonic signs of keratoconus. However, either Vogt's striae or a Fleischer's ring was observed in 68% of eyes, and either Vogt's striae, a Fleischer's ring, or corneal scarring was observed in 73% of eyes and more advanced disease (steeper average keratometric reading) was associated with a greater likelihood of Vogt's striae, Fleischer's ring, and/or corneal scarring.

Corneal hydrops occurs secondary to a rupture in Descemet's membrane in advanced keratoconus, allowing aqueous access to the corneal stroma, resulting in corneal edema at first and corneal scarring later (Plate 4). Although resolved corneal hydrops often can be accompanied by a flattening of the cornea, making rigid contact lens fitting easier, corneal hydrops is a poor prognostic sign if the contralateral eye is uninvolved; Fanta[49] has presented evidence suggesting that 40% of keratoconus patients suffering acute corneal hydrops will go on to develop hydrops in the other eye within 10 years. Patients with keratoconus and Down syndrome are known to have a higher than normal incidence of corneal hydrops, between 5% and 8%.

Fleischer's ring, appearing yellow-brown to olive-green in white light, represents hemosiderin deposits in the deep epithelium and presumably outlines the base of the cone. As the disease progresses, the ring becomes denser in its pigmentation, narrower, and may become a complete ring if it was partial earlier on. It is present in approximately 50% of cases. This prevalence may turn out to be higher with careful slit lamp examination of the corneal epithelium, including meticulous focusing on the epithelium and the employment of the cobalt blue filter to outline the iron visually.

Corneal scarring at or near the apex of the cone is characteristic of keratoconus, and its relationship to contact lens fitting method is a topic of some controversy.[50] Sometimes, elevated corneal scars ("proud nebulae") develop, and simple surgery to shave them off even with the corneal surface can allow contact lens wear again.[51] Not much is known about corneal scarring in keratoconus, its annual incidence, or how it relates to disease progression, but techniques are in development to document such scarring.[52]

Visually evident thinning at, or just below, the corneal apex is one sign of keratoconus. Although unable to define an absolute central pachometric value as diagnostic of keratoconus, Mandell and Polse[53] found a characteristic difference (at least 0.085 mm) between the central corneal thickness and the corneal thickness 35 degrees in the periphery. Corneal thickness may be within the normal range and is not one of the best diagnostic features, however.[54]

Other methods for diagnosing keratoconus utilize the peculiar light reflexes occurring from the geometry of the cornea. Poster and associates[55] have described an endothelial light reflex occurring at the cone's apex because of the increased posterior corneal curvature in this region. Shaw and associates[56] showed that viewing with the direct ophthalmoscope resulted in visualization of the outline of the cone as a honey or oil droplet against the red reflex of the fundus.

Rizzuti[57] has described a penlight test for keratoconus. When illuminating the cornea with a penlight from the temporal side of the cornea, focused anterior to the iris, light is sharply focused on the temporal side of the nasal limbus. A late sign of keratoconus on external examination is Munson's sign, where the lower lid angulates over the cone in downgaze.[58]

Keratoscopic Findings

Keratometric readings are typically steeper than normal, with irregular mires or mires that cannot be aligned. Inferior steepening can be evident on keratoscopic examination (Plate 5), but the presence of > 1.00 D of steepening seen with routine keratometry performed in the inferior cornea is a firm diagnostic sign.

Some clinicians emphasize the value of documented increases in keratometric curvature of the cornea over time in diagnosing early keratoconus. Lack of agreement between corneal toricity and refractive astigmatism is also a sign of early keratoconus, especially when accompanied by documented irregular astigmatism.

Recently, sophisticated corneal modeling systems have been used to characterize the topography of the disease and to assist in diagnosing early keratoconus.[40, 59–62] The advent of these computerized systems for the measurement of corneal topography has resulted in increased information about corneal shape in keratoconus. Topographic patterns include the classic inferior steepening but extend to include some corneas with steepening above the horizontal midline and others with flattening in the superior nasal quadrant.[61] A few cases of advancing surface irregularity are illustrated in Plates 5–9.

Investigators have touted corneal modeling as a tool for identifying subclinical keratoconus.[40, 59, 60, 63] However, it remains to be seen whether these "early" cases may represent keratoconus that never progresses beyond this early stage—representing some *forme fruste* or aborted form or variable expression of a keratoconus gene,[40] or whether these patients go on to develop classic keratoconus. Longitudinal studies of these patients are required to make this differentiation.

The reliability and validity of these devices has been only sporadically investigated,[64–66] and studies have yet to explore the reliability and validity of videokeratography findings for keratoconus corneas. For example, unanswered questions about topographic measurement with a corneal modeling device in keratoconus include: (1) Is the position of the corneal apex consistent between measurements? (2) Are the absolute values for corneal curvature consistent in the steep corneal areas and/or the normal corneal areas? (3) Is the overall pattern of corneal steepening, regardless of absolute values, consistent between measurements? (4) How dramatic a change in apex position, absolute curvature values, and topographic pattern is necessary to document disease progression?

Classification Schemes

There are many classification schemes for keratoconus. The most often described classification categories are the round, or nipple-shaped cone, and the oval, or sagging cone.[67,68] The round-cone type is smaller, has an apex that lies inferonasally, and is more amenable to rigid contact lens fitting. The oval cone is larger and centers infero-temporally. It often is associated with difficulty in contact lens application, anterior scarring, and episodes of acute corneal hydrops. However, specification of cone type, per se, is probably less important in contact lens application than cone location.

Impact on Patients

In addition to the visual compromise invariably present in keratoconus, optometrists and ophthalmologists who see a large number of keratoconus patients often report that these patients have personality disorders. Descriptive adjectives might include paranoid, anxious, compulsive, and somatic. Very few studies have examined this phenomenon in a rigorous way. Ridley[21] considered eye rubbing as a possible reaction to the emotional tension present in keratoconus and its visual compromise. Karseras and Ruben[20] had 75 patients with keratoconus and 231 normal controls complete a personality inventory and found no increased incidence of such psychoneuroses as anxiety, phobias, depression, obsession, and hysteria. Besançon and associates[69] interviewed 34 keratoconus patients at the time of admission for penetrating keratoplasty and found no specific constellation of psychotic symptoms but claimed a greater prevalence of neurologic and psychosomatic traits, without comparison to controls. Mannis et al.[70] used a personality questionnaire to compare keratoconus patients both to normal controls and to age-matched patients with chronic, nonkeratoconic eye disease. They found abnormal results on the same psychological scales (passive-aggressive, paranoid, hypomanic, disorganized thinking patterns, and substance abuse) in both the keratoconus and chronic eye disease patients. These studies, in the face of persistent clinical assertions that keratoconus patients have unique, difficult personalities, may not have found the appropriate psychological measuring rule for these possible personality abnormalities.

Progression

Keratoconus, after its initial onset somewhere between the second and third decades of life, progresses over the next 10 to 20 years, and its final severity differs across patients.[5] Some patients progress to the point of significant corneal thinning with visual needs still well managed with contact lenses, while others develop significantly scarred corneas. Typically, penetrating keratoplasty is performed in 10–20% of keratoconus cases and is successful 90–95% of the time in giving an optically clear cornea.[4, 7, 71]

There is good evidence that the classic slit lamp biomicroscopic signs (Vogt's striae, Fleischer's ring, and corneal scarring) of keratoconus are associated with disease severity when severity is specified by keratometry. Patients are more likely to have at least one and more likely to have two or more of these signs with increasing disease severity.[7] The Collaborative Longitudinal Evaluation of Keratoconus (CLEK) Study has enrolled a projected 1,210 keratoconus patients in 1995–1996 and will provide a great deal of information about disease progression in keratoconus when the study finishes in 2004.

Spectacle Correction

Because the corneal curvature changes in keratoconus, with rare exception, result in myopia and astigmatism, patients require some type of visual correction from the earliest stages. Most practitioners rely on spectacles in the early course of the disease. Limitations on spectacle correction in keratoconus include: (1) high amounts of corneal toricity and resultant refractive astigmatism, the correction of which is not tolerable in spectacle form; (2) changing refractive error, either diurnally or from week to week, for which spectacles cannot be adequately prescribed; (3) inadequacy of visual acuity with spectacles because of uncorrected irregular astigmatism; and (4) anisometropia present as a result of the asymmetric nature of the disease. Even given these problems, however, spectacles are the first form of optical management of the disease, especially in its early stages. They can provide surprisingly good visual acuity,[7] and subjective refraction is reasonably repeatable.[72] Contact lenses typically can correct irregular astigmatism and improve visual acuity beyond the level of spectacles but should be reserved for those patients in whom spectacles are no longer adequate.

Rigid Contact Lens Correction

The use of rigid contact lenses, both before and since the introduction of gas permeable materials, has been the mainstay of the optical management of keratoconus. These lenses, manufactured in a large variety of unique designs, provide a regular surface over the cornea and allow the intervening fluid lens to correct the corneal astigmatism adequately in most cases.

Certainly a rigid gas permeable contact lens allows for a far more uniform refracting surface than the irregular astigmatic surface of the keratoconic cornea. The local irregularities of the (often) stained and (sometimes) raised epithelial lesion are filled in by the tears behind the rigid gas permeable lens. However, the lacrimal lens only eliminates about 90% of the cornea's astigmatic error due to the index difference between the tears and cornea.[73] Corneal scarring and epithelial staining diffuse light and result in worse low contrast visual acuity. The rigid gas permeable lens may also further distort the cornea. A flat or steep fit may cause wrinkling of the epithelium, and one cannot rule out that a very flat fit may decrease axial length.

In addition, although lenses often position over the apex of the displaced ectatic area, rigid lenses eliminate the difficulties associated with this displacement by also superimposing the visual axis. Rigid lens fitting in keratoconus is, however, by no means simple. Numerous lenses are often required, even for an initial fitting, and achieving an adequate cornea-lens fitting relationship with reasonable vision becomes more difficult as the disease progresses. Although most practitioners who fit a large variety of keratoconus patients have their preferences for lens design,[50, 67, 74–86] most practicing clinicians still find each keratoconus patient a trial-and-error experience. Some common lens designs are summarized in Table 1. Refitting is often required at relatively frequent intervals.

Virtually all literature reports on contact lens fitting in keratoconus are anecdotal in the sense that they represent retrospective

Table 1. Keratoconus Contact Lens Designs and Trial Lens Sets

Lens Design	Diameter	Optic Zone	Peripheral Curvatures
Soper	8.5	7.0	7.50/.25, 8.40/.10, 9.10/.20, 13/.20
McGuire	8.6	6.0	SCR* = BCR + 0.5 mm, TCR* = BCR + 1.5 mm
	9.1	6.5	PCR* = BCR + 4.5 mm
	9.5	7.0	similar for all diameters
Rose K	8.7	varies with aspheric base curve	
CLEK	8.6	6.5	8.5 SCR, 11.0 PCR/.2
SoftPerm	14.3 with 8.0 styrene rigid central portion		
Flexlens Tricurve	14.0 (Note: these lenses have 0.40 to 0.28 CT for correcting irregular astigmatism)		
Harrison	15.0		
Piggyback	14.5	10.2 mm (or as specified) cut out for rigid gas permeable lens	

* SCR = Secondary curve radius.
  TCR = Tertiary curve radius.
  PCR = Peripheral curve radius.

data on a clinical population of keratoconus patients. Nonetheless, these studies do provide information on the large variety of lens types that have been utilized successfully in the management of keratoconus, although success rates must be viewed with some skepticism because of lack of controls, possible bias in patients selected for fitting, and varying definitions of what constitutes a successful contact lens fitting in a keratoconus patient (Table 2).

The studies outlined in Table 2 report variable success rates, although most are on the order of 80%, judged in some cases by the absence of adverse corneal physiologic effects and in others by visu-

Table 2. Summary of Studies on Rigid Lens Correction in Keratoconus

Author(s), Year	No. of Eyes	No. of Patients	Lens Type
Retrospective			
Gould, 1970	NS	44	PMMA, 7–8 mm in diameter
Soper and Jarrett, 1972	178	NS	Soper Cone
Gasset and Lobo, 1975	60	43	Dura-T
Mobilia and Foster, 1979	96	56	Polycon
Raber, 1983	23	19	CAB Soper Cone
Lembach and Keates, 1984	22	20	Silcon aspheric
Cohen and Parlato, 1986	123	NS	Polycon II
Kastl et al., 1987	83	64	PMMA, CAB
Prospective			
Korb et al., 1982	14	7	Polycon; randomized flat vs. steep
Maguen et al., 1983	31	17	Polycon (previous contact lens failures)

al acuity or wearing time and comfort. By and large, it seems that whatever lens a particular clinician becomes comfortable with and adept at using works well in that clinician's hands.

Rigid Contact Lenses and the Etiology of Keratoconus

Numerous authors have reported keratoconus occurring in patients wearing rigid contact lenses and have implied that the lenses were instrumental in the causation of the disease.[15, 17, 18, 22, 87–89] Only two studies have attempted to define this association in a large group of patients. Gasset et al.[15] compared 162 diagnosed keratoconus patients with 1,248 soft contact lens patients and found a high incidence of rigid contact lens wear that preceded the keratoconus (26.5%). This comparison of a retrospective group of cases (patients with keratoconus) with a prospective group of controls (soft contact lens wearers) has been severely criticized for its poor epidemiological methodology[90, 91] and can certainly be ignored.

Brightbill and Stainer[88] examined 120 keratoconus patients and found a positive history of contact lens wear prior to diagnosis in 17.5%, but had no control group for comparison. Eggink and associates[6] examined a large group of keratoconus patients in the Netherlands and found that 5.9% of them reported a history of diagnosis during rigid contact lens wear. Macsai and coworkers[92] compared their patients who were first diagnosed with keratoconus to those who wore rigid contact lenses prior to the diagnosis of keratoconus and found that the initial rigid lens wearers had less severe keratoconus: they were younger and had flatter keratometric readings. In general, since rigid contact lens application is a treatment for keratoconus and since early keratoconus can be subtle to detect, a causative relationship between the two may be impossible to ascertain, even if it exists.

Rigid Contact Lens Fitting Methods

The major rigid lens fitting techniques in keratoconus, as succinctly described by Korb et al.,[50] are: (1) *apical bearing,* with primary lens support on the apex of the cornea (Plate 10), where the central optic zone of the lens actually touches or bears on the central corneal epithelium;[77] (2) *apical clearance,* with lens support and bearing directed off the apex and onto the paracentral cornea (Plate 11), with clearance of the apex of the cornea;[86] and (3) divided support or *three-point touch,* with lens support and bearing shared between the corneal apex and the paracentral cornea (Plate 12).

Typically, an apical bearing fit is the easiest to achieve in keratoconus. Almost all rigid contact lenses touch the apex of the cone unless steps are taken to alleviate the bearing or actually to clear the corneal apex. In three-point touch, although possibly viewed as a variant of apical touch, the contact lens fitter attempts to minimize the touch on the corneal apex by steepening the lens centrally and allowing the peripheral cornea to show areas of light touch, thereby minimizing trauma to all areas of the cornea. The major disadvantage of apical touch is the possibility of epithelial trauma and the inducement of corneal scarring. Its advantages include the possibility of superior acuity,[93] although more exhaustive studies have not borne out this observation.[94]

In lenses fitted with an apical clearance technique, trauma to the central cornea and epithelium is presumably minimized. Wearing time may be lessened relative to lenses supported more by the central cornea, but rigorous, well-controlled studies have not been performed to verify this.

One study best addresses the issues relative to the best fitting technique to apply for keratoconus. Korb et al.[50] performed a fitting study on 14 eyes of 7 keratoconus patients that conformed to a rigorous set of entry criteria. They "semirandomized" the eyes to either a large and flat or small and steep lens (i.e., in half the patients, the more advanced eye was fitted with the flat lens and in the other half, the less advanced eye was fitted with the flat lens). Within a 12-month period, 4 of the 7 eyes fitted with the flat-fitting method developed corneal scarring; within the same period of time, none of the eyes fitted steep developed any scarring. Potential confounding variables that were not discussed included the influence of contact lens diameter, the possibility of differential wearing time, and the potential for increased staining with the silicone/acrylate material used, relative to other polymers. Nonetheless, this study still introduces the possibility that the current standard of care, wherein the corneal apex typically supports some of the weight of the contact lens across the cornea,[7] may, in fact, result in some proportion of the corneal scarring observed in keratoconus.

Specific Rigid Lens Fitting Rationale

Contact lens fitting in keratoconus, although often discussed,[50, 67, 71, 74, 76–83, 85, 86] is difficult to specify. The cornea with keratoconus can vary with respect to any combination of the following factors: (1) cone position, (2) cone size, (3) degree of induced myopia, (4) amount of corneal toricity, (5) steepness of keratometric readings, (6) corneal topographic profile, (7) disease progression with respect to both degree and rate, (8) achievement of contact lens–corrected visual acuity, and (9) contact lens tolerance. As such, one recipe to be applied to the fitting of all keratoconus patients cannot be written, but fitting *pearls* are often helpful. Some laboratories will loan trial lens sets to practitioners.

The contact lens practitioner needs to be extraordinarily creative in his or her lens design for keratoconus. The objective is to provide adequate vision with acceptable corneal tissue tolerance for an adequate number of hours of wear per day. Several fitting sets should be available for trial fitting use, such as those specified by Mandell[95] and Korb et al.[50] These lenses, with their smaller diameters (8.6 mm), can be used to achieve an apical clearance or three-point touch fluorescein pattern, if such a fit is appropriate for a given cornea. The larger-diameter lenses (to 9.2 mm) lend themselves well to three-point touch or apical touch fitting methods and can be helpful in an inferiorly displaced cone. The choice of fitting philosophy and, therefore, lens choice is often one of necessity. Although the practitioner may actually intend to fit a lens so that it clears the corneal apex, good comfort and vision may be achieved with a lens that lightly touches the central cornea. On other keratoconic corneas, the apical clearance fitting pattern may be achieved easily. Toric base curve lenses typically are avoided because the corneal toricity is not regular.

Aspheric lenses, such as VFL II and Ellip-See-Con (Conform Contact Lenses, Norfolk, VA), among others, have been used successfully and described in great detail by other authors.[79, 96] These lenses generally are fitted steep in relation to corneal curvature, and lens diameter is dependent on the base curve-eccentricity value relationship of the lens (i.e., if the eccentricity value of a given lens needs to be increased, then the base curve would be ordered steeper with a smaller overall diameter, to maintain proper edge lift).[96]

In both diagnostic fitting and evaluating the fit of a dispensed lens, the malleability of the keratoconic cornea is important. Any rigid lens placed on a keratoconic cornea should be allowed to equilibrate on the eye for a minimum of 10 to 20 minutes. Often, dispensed lenses fit differently (more or less successfully) at a one-week follow-up visit than they do initially.

Diagnostic lenses with known peripheral curve systems must be used. If a decision must be made about altering the specified peripheral curves, it is better to err on the shorter radius of curvature, or steep, side. This allows the practitioner to modify the peripheral system of the lens in the office by flattening the curves.

In-office modification of keratoconus lenses is imperative. In addition to peripheral curve modification as mentioned above, edges frequently require small or moderate modifications. Peripheral curves often have to be blended to a greater degree than the laboratory supplies them. Because keratoconus patients frequently have difficulty with subjective overrefractions or diagnostic lenses are quite different in power than the final power ordered, small in-office additions of minus power may be necessary.

The retinoscope is a valuable tool both for diagnosing keratoconus and for managing it with rigid contact lenses. In attempting to overrefract a patient whose sensitivity to blur may be in a 1.00 to 2.00 D range, time, effort, and frustration often can be minimized by first performing a retinoscopic overrefraction.

Refitting the successful keratoconus patient should be initiated with great restraint. The keratoconus patient who wears lenses 14 hours per day without discomfort and has good vision but would like two more hours of wearing time is not a good candidate for refitting. Neither is the patient who has 20/25 acuity but complains of inadequate vision. The known decrements in vision in keratoconus are not typically fully eliminated with rigid contact lens correction.[42, 44, 45]

Painstaking, up-to-date records should be maintained on each keratoconus patient's lens(es) and any modifications that have been performed on them, so that rapid, efficient duplication in the event of a lost or damaged lens is possible.

Rigid Lens Fitting Procedure

Information on the diagnosis of and fitting methods for keratoconus has been presented. A specific procedure to facilitate fitting or refitting the keratoconus patient follows.

Keratometry

Although keratometric readings may be of limited usefulness in fitting keratoconus patients, they can assist in initial trial lens selection and in documenting disease progression. The keratometric range should be extended as necessary.[95] The protocol used in the Collaborative Longitudinal Evaluation of Keratoconus (CLEK) Study is as follows:

If the patient's cornea is steeper than 52.00 D (i.e., off the scale) in either meridian, the range of the keratometer will need to be extended as follows:

(1) Apply a +1.25 D lens to the keratometer (objective side).

(2) Table 3 should be consulted to convert the readings with the +1.25 D lens in place to actual readings.

(3) If the patient's cornea is off the scale of the keratometer in either meridian with the +1.25 D lens in place, steps 1–2 above should be repeated with the +2.25 D lens in place, consulting Table 4 for the conversion of the drum reading to the actual reading.

(4) If the patient's cornea is off the scale of the keratometer in either meridian with the +2.25 D lens in place, record the keratometric meridian in that meridian as "> 68.30."

Refraction

Careful refraction is mandatory. Patients with keratoconus often have unpredictably good best-corrected visual acuity. High amounts of cylinder, frequently at an increasingly oblique axis, are sometimes found. Retinoscopic and keratometric results are an excellent starting point for determining the subjective refraction. Careful refinement of

Table 3. Extending the Range of the Keratometer with a +1.25 D Lens.

Drum reading	Corneal Power in Diopters	Drum reading	Corneal Power in Diopters
43.00	50.13	47.62	55.53
43.12	50.28	47.75	55.67
43.25	50.43	47.87	55.82
43.37	50.57	48.00	55.96
43.50	50.72	48.12	56.11
43.62	50.86	48.25	56.25
43.75	51.01	48.37	56.40
43.87	51.15	48.50	56.55
44.00	51.30	48.62	56.69
44.12	51.45	48.75	56.84
44.25	51.59	48.87	56.98
44.37	51.74	49.00	57.13
44.50	51.88	49.12	57.27
44.62	52.03	49.25	57.42
44.75	52.17	49.37	57.57
44.87	52.32	49.50	57.71
45.00	52.47	49.62	57.86
45.12	52.61	49.75	58.00
45.25	52.76	49.87	58.15
45.37	52.90	50.00	58.29
45.50	53.05	50.12	58.44
45.62	53.19	50.25	58.59
45.75	53.34	50.37	58.73
45.87	53.49	50.50	58.88
46.00	53.63	50.62	59.02
46.12	53.78	50.75	59.17
46.25	53.92	50.87	59.32
46.37	54.07	51.00	59.46
46.50	54.21	51.12	59.61
46.62	54.36	51.25	59.75
46.75	54.51	51.37	59.90
46.87	54.65	51.50	60.04
47.00	54.80	51.62	60.19
47.12	54.94	51.75	60.34
47.25	55.09	51.87	60.48
47.37	55.23	52.00	60.63
47.50	55.38		

Table 4. Extending the Range of the Keratometer with a +2.25 D Lens.

Drum reading	Corneal Power in Diopters	Drum reading	Corneal Power in Diopters
43.00	56.43	47.62	62.53
43.12	56.59	47.75	62.69
43.25	56.76	47.87	62.86
43.37	56.92	48.00	63.02
43.50	57.09	48.12	63.19
43.62	57.25	48.25	63.35
43.75	57.42	48.37	63.52
43.87	57.58	48.50	63.68
44.00	57.75	48.62	63.85
44.12	57.91	48.75	64.01
44.25	58.08	48.87	64.18
44.37	58.24	49.00	64.34
44.50	58.41	49.12	64.51
44.62	58.57	49.25	64.67
44.75	58.74	49.37	64.84
44.87	58.90	49.50	65.00
45.00	59.07	49.62	65.17
45.12	59.23	49.75	65.33
45.25	59.40	49.87	65.50
45.37	59.56	50.00	65.66
45.50	59.73	50.12	65.83
45.62	59.89	50.25	65.99
45.75	60.06	50.37	66.16
45.87	60.22	50.50	66.32
46.00	60.38	50.62	66.49
46.12	60.55	50.75	66.65
46.25	60.71	50.87	66.81
46.37	60.88	51.00	66.98
46.50	61.04	51.12	67.14
46.62	61.21	51.25	67.31
46.75	61.37	51.37	67.47
46.87	61.54	51.50	67.64
47.00	61.70	51.62	67.80
47.12	61.87	51.75	67.97
47.25	62.03	51.87	68.13
47.37	62.20	52.00	68.30
47.50	62.36		

PLATE 1. Apical corneal thinning and apical corneal scarring typical of keratoconus.

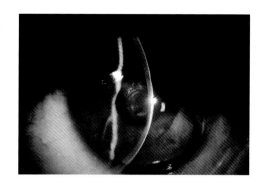

PLATE 2. Obliquely oriented Vogt's striae in the posterior stroma.

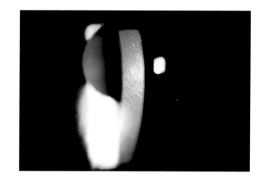

PLATE 3. Fleischer's ring at the base of the ectatic area.

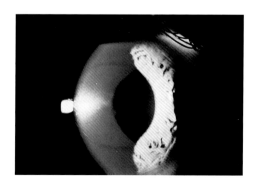

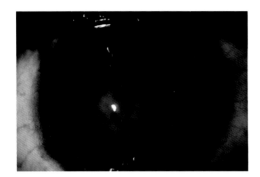

PLATE 4. Keratoconic cornea following an episode of corneal hydrops.

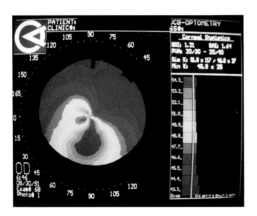

PLATE 5. Inferior corneal steepening characteristic of early keratoconus.

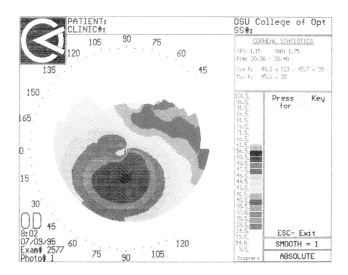

PLATE 6. This corneal map illustrates a typical inferior corneal area of ectasia, which is common in mild keratoconus. In this case the "apical" curvature, according to the map, is 56.5 diopters.

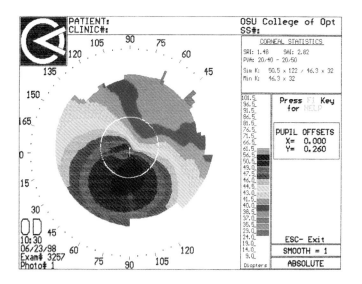

PLATE 7. This map is from the same eye as that depicted in Plate 6 (nearly three years later) and illustrates a larger area of ectasia. (Mandell [1992] has demonstrated that if one positions the corneal apex to correspond with the optic axis of the videokeratoscope, the apical curvature is much steeper and the cornea now appears to be regular with very high eccentricity.)

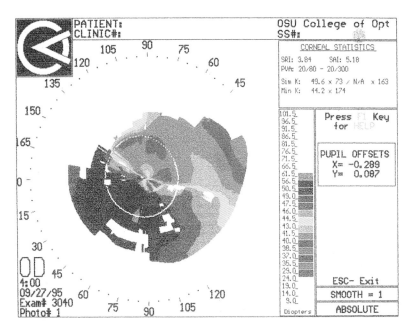

PLATE 8. This map illustrates a wider area of ectasia than depicted in Plates 6 or 7. The missing areas in the map illustrate corneal surface irregularity, which the video-keratoscope did not process. This irregularity may be from epithelial staining, local surface roughness, or poor cornea-tear interface wetting. Some videokeratoscope systems will "smooth" this irregularity.

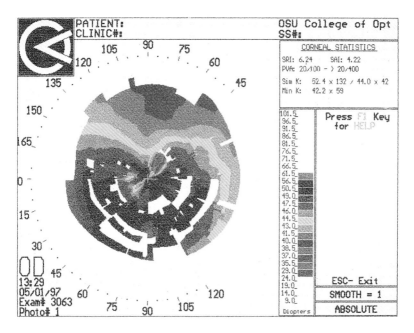

PLATE 9. This map illustrates an even wider area of ectasia that encompasses nearly the entire inferior area of the map.

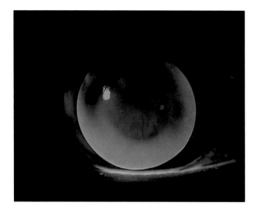

PLATE 10. Apical touch fit with maximum acceptable edge lift.

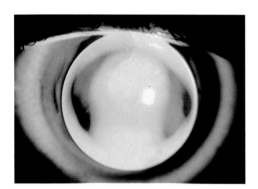

PLATE 11. Apical clearance fit with good edge lift.

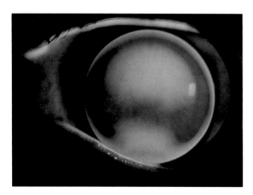

PLATE 12. Three-point touch with inadequate edge lift.

PLATE 13. Rigid contact lens on a keratoconic cornea. The base curve of the lens is 7.55 mm. Photograph courtesy of Timothy B. Edrington, O.D. M.S.

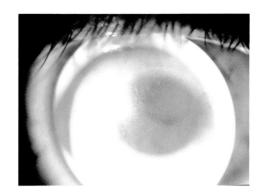

PLATE 14. Rigid contact lens on the same keratoconic cornea as that pictured in Plate 13. The base curve of the lens is 7.42 mm. Photograph courtesy of Timothy B. Edrington, O.D. M.S.

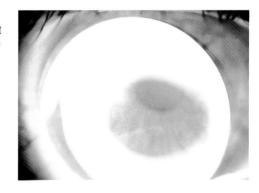

PLATE 15. Rigid contact lens on the same keratoconic cornea as that pictured in Plate 13. The base curve of the lens is 7.31 mm. Photograph courtesy of Timothy B. Edrington, O.D. M.S.

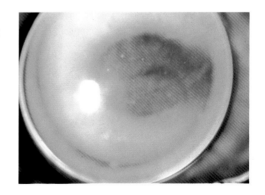

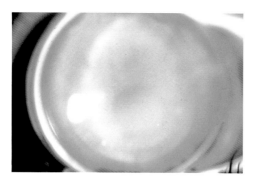

PLATE 16. Rigid contact lens on the same keratoconic cornea as that pictured in Plate 13. The base curve of the lens is 6.72 mm. Photograph courtesy of Timothy B. Edrington, O.D. M.S.

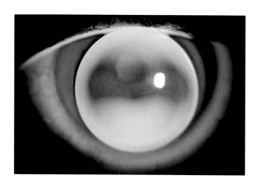

PLATE 17. This plate illustrates moderate edge lift at 12:00 and acceptable edge lift at 3:00 and 9:00. At 6:00 the edge lift is moderate to excessive. If comfort is acceptable and the lens does not dislodge, this is very acceptable edge lift.

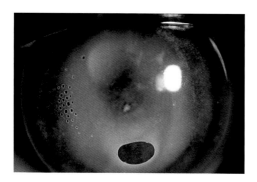

PLATE 18. At dispensing this lens illustrated acceptable to minimal edge lift. Six hours later, there are bubbles trapped behind the lens, and there is minimal to no edge lift. Although the edge lift can be increased by flattening the peripheral curves and decreasing optic zone size, this will result in increased apical touch.

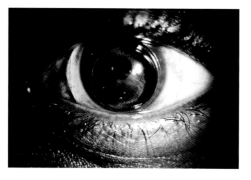

PLATE 19. Piggyback lens system with a countersunk hydrogel lens carrier.

cylinder axis and avoidance of overminusing are necessary. Accurate refraction provides a baseline best visual acuity without contact lenses, which serves as a reference point for expected contact lens corrected acuity. Contact lens corrected acuity should be at least as good as that achieved with spectacles. Subjective refraction results are often prescribed, either as back-up spectacles for patients who wear contact lenses, or as the primary mode of correction for patients who cannot wear contact lenses.[7]

Trial Lens Fitting
A trial lens fitting is vital in fitting rigid lenses on patients with keratoconus. There is no "formula" approach for predicting a proper lens fit. The initial trial lens should be chosen with a base curve that either splits the two keratometric readings or is equal to the steep corneal curvature. If the patient has never worn contact lenses, instillation of a topical corneal anesthetic may be helpful in obtaining an accurate visual acuity measurement and assessment of the fluorescein pattern without excessive tearing.

Fluorescein Pattern Analysis
The ideal keratoconic fluorescein pattern depends on the lens design chosen. The central pattern will depend on which of the contact lens fitting methods outlined above one is trying to achieve. The peripheral curve should be flat enough to allow a reservoir of tears to collect without allowing excessive edge lift and lens dislocation. This combination aids in tear interchange and movement.

To analyze the fit, the fluorescein pattern should be divided into two areas: the central portion, including the entire area under the optic zone, and the peripheral zone. Each area should be analyzed separately. The location and amount of bearing should be observed. (Note in Plates 13–16, showing progressively steeper base curves on the same cornea, that the fluorescein pattern may not change appreciably from lens to lens if the base curve change between lenses is relatively small.) If there is central bearing, the lens should be steepened if an apical clearance pattern is desired.[50]

If pooling in the periphery is absent, the peripheral systems should be flatter (Plates 17–18). If there is insufficient lens movement and excessive bearing in the area of the secondary curves, then the secondary curve is too steep, preventing lens movement. Absence of fluorescein in the secondary or peripheral area can be due to the peripheral lens "seal-off." Horizontally, edge lift may be just adequate, while inferiorly, edge lift may be on the high end of acceptable. Presence of any air bubbles under the lens should be carefully noted as to location, size, and persistence. A central air bubble may mean that the lens is too steep. Paracentral air bubbles, on the other hand, may mean that the optic zone is too large. A good rule of thumb is for the optic zone to approximately equal the base curve. Small optic zones on the steepest lenses may unfortunately result in flare to achieve the best fit.

Corneal apex position relative to the trial lens should be determined. Generally, the lower the apex, the larger the diameter of the lens required for centration. A low-riding lens may be too flat or too small. A larger lens may be required for centration. In attempting to fit a larger lens, a lid attachment fit is desirable; however the peripheral system must be flat enough to prevent paracentral seal-off resulting in decreased movement and inadequate tear exchange.

Each trial lens should be allowed to settle on the eye for an appropriate amount of time (approximately 20 minutes) prior to evaluation. Keratoconic corneas are very pliable, and in the case of a previous wearer of flat lenses, the degree of corneal molding can be marked.

Successive trial lens overrefractions should be compared, and the total power of each system should be approximately equal. This is important for evaluating the consistency of the diagnostic lenses, their optical performance on the eye, and the patient's consistency during subjective overrefraction.

Once an adequate fit is achieved, a manufacturing laboratory must be chosen that will make the lens according to specifications.

Some laboratories have a standard keratoconic lens design, but these lenses are often too steep peripherally. If the ordered lens looks different from the diagnostic trial lens, in-office or laboratory modification will be necessary. It is extremely important that an individual trial lens set be manufactured according to specifications to insure a standardization factor for comparison, both during fitting and as a check against ordered lenses. A gas permeable material of medium DK (12-60) is recommended. This allows ample oxygen and is less prone to warpage and dryness.

CLEK Study Fitting Protocol

Recently, the CLEK Study has published a standardized protocol for fitting keratoconus patients based on sagittal height.[97] Parameters for the CLEK diagnostic keratoconus fitting set were determined as follows:

1. Base curve radii were selected to encompass the corneal sagittal heights for mild to moderate keratoconus patients. Increments of 0.05 mm were chosen to increase the fitting sensitivity.

2. Contact lens powers were chosen to provide low minus over-refractions for the majority of mild to moderate keratoconus patients.

3. The overall diameter was set at 8.6 mm to provide an interpalpebral fit in which the lens positions over the apex of the conical area of the cornea.

4. The optic zone diameter was standardized at 6.5 mm to minimize areas of tear pooling and debris accumulation under the optic zone of the lens.

5. The secondary curve radius ranged from 8.00 to 8.25 mm in order to obtain average peripheral clearance. Corneal curvatures beyond the cone are similar to corneal curvatures of nonkeratoconus patients. Therefore, secondary curve radii appropriate for nonkeratoconus RGP contact lens fitting are indicated.

6. The peripheral or third curve radius for the tricurve fitting lenses was set at 11.00 mm with a width of 0.20 mm. This curve was selected not only to be a fitting curve, but also to start the posterior edge treatment.

7. Center thicknesses were calculated such that an edge thickness of approximately 0.10 mm was maintained for each trial lens. Center thicknesses are thicker than cosmetic RGP lenses of similar power because of the flatter secondary curve to base curve relationship.

8. Diagnostic lenses were fabricated in polymethylmethacrylate (PMMA) material. PMMA was chosen because of its machinability, dimensional stability, durability, and low cost. Lenses for patients can be manufactured in any rigid lens material.

The contact lens practitioner determined the steep keratometry reading, converted it to mm, and referred to Table 5 for selection of the initial trial lens from the CLEK Study diagnostic contact lens set.

For example:

Keratometry readings:	48.50/51.50 @ 115
Average keratometry value:	50.00 D = 6.75 mm
Select initial trial lens	No. 23

The initial trial lens was applied to the subject's eye and allowed to settle for 10 minutes prior to analysis of the fluorescein pattern.

If the initial trial lens was judged to be flat, the next higher numbered (steeper) trial lens was applied to the eye for fluorescein pattern evaluation. This procedure was repeated until a definite apical clearance pattern was achieved. Therefore, the endpoint of the contact lens fitting procedure was the flattest lens in the trial lens set that exhibited a definite apical clearance fluorescein pattern such that the sagittal depth of the base curve chord diameter was greater than the sagittal depth of the cornea for the same chord diameter. The base

Table 5. CLEK Study Keratoconus Diagnostic Lens Set. (Edrington, et al., 1996).

All diagnostic contact lenses are PMMA with a third curve radius of 11.00 mm and a third curve width of 0.2 mm. The lenses are lightly blended, and the center thickness is 0.13 mm.

Lens No.	Inside Sagittal Depth Under Optic Zone (mm)	Base Curve in mm (Diopters)	Power (D)	Overall Diameter/ Optic Zone Diameter (mm)	Secondary Curve Radius (mm)
1	0.704	7.85 (42.99)	−3.00	8.6/6.5	8.25
2	0.709	7.80 (43.27)	−4.00	8.6/6.5	8.25
3	0.714	7.75 (43.55)	−3.00	8.6/6.5	8.25
4	0.719	7.70 (43.83)	−4.00	8.6/6.5	8.25
5	0.725	7.65 (44.12)	−3.00	8.6/6.5	8.25
6	0.730	7.60 (44.41)	−4.00	8.6/6.5	8.25
7	0.735	7.55 (44.70)	−5.00	8.6/6.5	8.25
8	0.741	7.50 (45.00)	−4.00	8.6/6.5	8.25
9	0.746	7.45 (45.30)	−5.00	8.6/6.5	8.25
10	0.752	7.40 (45.61)	−6.00	8.6/6.5	8.25
11	0.757	7.35 (45.92)	−4.00	8.6/6.5	8.25
12	0.763	7.30 (46.23)	−5.00	8.6/6.5	8.25
13	0.769	7.25 (46.55)	−6.00	8.6/6.5	8.25
14	0.775	7.20 (46.87)	−5.00	8.6/6.5	8.25
15	0.781	7.15 (47.20)	−6.00	8.6/6.5	8.25
16	0.787	7.10 (47.54)	−7.00	8.6/6.5	8.25
17	0.794	7.05 (47.87)	−5.00	8.6/6.5	8.25
18	0.800	7.00 (48.21)	−6.00	8.6/6.5	8.25
19	0.807	6.95 (48.56)	−7.00	8.6/6.5	8.25
20	0.813	6.90 (48.91)	−6.00	8.6/6.5	8.25
21	0.820	6.85 (49.27)	−7.00	8.6/6.5	8.25
22	0.827	6.80 (49.63)	−8.00	8.6/6.5	8.25
23	0.834	6.75 (50.00)	−6.00	8.6/6.5	8.25
24	0.842	6.70 (50.37)	−7.00	8.6/6.5	8.25
25	0.848	6.65 (50.75)	−8.00	8.6/6.5	8.25
26	0.856	6.60 (51.14)	−6.00	8.6/6.5	8.00
27	0.865	6.55 (51.53)	−7.00	8.6/6.5	8.00
28	0.870	6.50 (51.92)	−8.00	8.6/6.5	8.00
29	0.879	6.45 (52.33)	−7.00	8.6/6.5	8.00
30	0.886	6.40 (52.73)	−8.00	8.6/6.5	8.00
31	0.895	6.35 (53.15)	−9.00	8.6/6.5	8.00
32	0.903	6.30 (53.57)	−7.00	8.6/6.5	8.00

curve radius of this lens was referred to as the "First Definite Apical Clearance Lens."

If the initial trial lens was judged to be steep centrally, the next lower numbered (flatter) trial lens in Table 5 was applied to the cornea for fluorescein pattern evaluation. This procedure was repeated until a definite apical touch or three-point touch was achieved.[98]

Hydrogel Contact Lens Correction

The use of hydrogel contact lenses in keratoconus may be indicated in two distinct situations. The first is during the early stages of keratoconus, when the apical protrusion and resulting irregular astigmatism are subtle and soft contact lenses can correct the myopia refractive error. The second is in later stages of the disease. Several authors have reported adequate vision with soft lens correction with and without spectacle overcorrection. Specific lens types are seldom discussed, although Koliopoulos and Tragakis[99] and Tragakis and Brown[100] used several different lenses and report visual acuity of 20/50 or better in 71 of 96 eyes fitted. Specialized soft lenses for keratoconus are available. These lenses correct the keratoconus due to lens thickness (averaging 0.4 to 0.5 mm thick). These lenses are generally used as an end-stage option, as they are more likely to result in edema and neovascularization secondary to the reduced oxygen transmissibility of these thick lenses.

Beyond custom soft toric contact lenses for early keratoconus and using common spherical soft contact lenses with rigid gas permeable lenses over them (a piggyback system), there are special soft contact lenses made by Paragon Vision Sciences' Flexlens Products (Englewood, CO). Flexlens tricurve keratoconus lenses have center thicknesses ranging from 0.40 to 0.45 mm and are available in base curves from 6.00 to 10.00 mm and diameters from 10.0 to 16.0 mm. Powers range from +30.00 to –30.00 D.

Piggyback and Hybrid Contact Lens Systems

In the late stages of prekeratoplasty keratoconus, a rigid gas permeable lens used over a hydrogel lens (a piggyback lens system) may improve comfort and the corneal surface regularity.[101] Its use is typically reserved for cases in which the apical corneal epithelium continually abrades with rigid contact lens wear, and only 1–2% of patients enrolled in the Collaborative Longitudinal Evaluation of Keratoconus (CLEK) Study wear this modality.[35] The underlying hydrogel lens acts as a bandage lens to prevent trauma to the epithelium from the rigid lens. These include an ultrathin hydrogel, a high plus hydrogel with steep central anterior curve, or a countersunk hydrogel with a groove cut slightly larger than the diameter of the rigid lens (Plate 19). The ultrathin hydrogel is the simplest option, providing higher oxygen transmissibility centrally under the rigid lens. Both the high plus lens and the countersunk lens attempt to improve rigid lens centration, potentially sacrificing oxygen transmissibility in the process.

Flexlens piggyback lenses have base curves ranging from 6.00 to 11.00 mm, diameters from 12.5 to 16.0 mm, and an anterior cutout for the rigid gas permeable lens can be made from 6.5 to 13.5 mm in diameter. The cutout is made 1 mm larger than the rigid gas permeable lens. For example, a 9.0-mm diameter rigid gas permeable lens would be ordered for a 10.00-mm cutout. The initial rigid gas permeable lens base curve is determined by performing keratometry over a well-fitted soft piggyback lens.

Specific fitting guidelines are difficult to outline, as the fit of the lens depends so heavily on the individual response of a particular eye and cornea. However, several points are important. Achieving adequate movement of the carrier hydrogel lens should be paramount, because doing so improves both comfort and debris removal capabilities. The rigid lens used prior to the piggyback fitting may be too steep and a flatter lens must be fitted and dispensed to eliminate central air bubbles trapped between the two lenses. The use of high molecular weight fluorescein is of limited usefulness here. Care systems must be chosen for their compatibility with both lens types. If possible, the use of saline as a wetting agent for both lenses eliminates any potential for preservative collection in the soft lens. If hydrogen peroxide systems are used, the rigid lens should be stored overnight in an appropriate rigid lens soaking solution. Both lenses can, and should be, routinely enzymatically cleaned. If piggyback lens systems fail, it typically is because of corneal edema or inconvenience to the patient in terms of lens handling and care.

Zadnik and Mannis[102] have reported that the Saturn II lens (a one-piece lens with a rigid center and a hydrogel skirt) may also provide improved comfort when rigid gas permeable lenses are uncomfortable, but only a small number of keratoconus patients wear such lenses. Because of its low oxygen transmissibility, the Saturn II (now called Softperm) lens is a lens of last resort for use in keratoconus and can produce marked vascularization, a finding atypical in keratoconus. Wearing time should be limited with this lens due to the overwear syndrome that can result from the induced hypoxia.

Gas Permeable Scleral Lenses

Scleral lenses have occupied a place in the management of keratoconus since the late 1800s, yet in recent years the use of this lens design has been extremely limited. A number of factors contributed to the demise of scleral lenses. The most significant of these was the corneal hypoxia that inevitably accompanied the use of polymethylmethacrylate scleral lenses despite numerous methods of ventilation (slots, fenestrations, channels, and truncations).

With the development of highly oxygen permeable polymers, corneal hypoxia has been greatly reduced.[103] This has provided an opportunity to re-evaluate the clinical applications of scleral lenses. Oxygen permeable polymers have been used clinically in the form of preformed or lathed oxygen permeable scleral lenses for keratoconus, aphakia, high refractive errors, and ocular surface disease.[104,][105] Because the highly oxygen permeable polymers are crosslinked, molding of gas permeable scleral lenses is not practical.[106]

Both fenestrated and nonventilated gas permeable scleral lenses have been described for the management of keratoconus. The use of fenestrations requires on-site modification equipment and skills to control the positioning and movement of air intrusion into the retrolens tear compartment through the fenestration. The size and continual movement of the air bubble created by the fenestration are extremely critical in minimizing the desiccating effects of the air on the corneal surface. Nonventilated lenses maintain a fluid compartment and exclude air intrusion into the retrolens space, thus liberalizing the tolerances for fitting the lens and minimizing the need for on-site modification.

Scleral lenses possess unique properties. Because they are supported by the scleral surface, centration can be achieved independent of the amount of corneal distortion. In addition, the lens vaults the corneal surface, eliminating any mechanical friction between the back surface of the lens and the cornea. These properties can be exploited in the management of keratoconus when more traditional strategies fail.

As previously discussed, contact lens failure in keratoconus results in penetrating keratoplasty and is usually the result of corneal contact lens intolerance or poor visual acuity.[1] Apical swirl staining, central corneal abrasions, fragile epithelium over elevated scarring, and unstable contact lenses may result in poor tolerance of a corneal lens. If refitting with a corneal lens design does not improve the contact lens tolerance, a gas permeable scleral lens may provide a stable, centered lens that by design has no contact with the corneal surface. This may delay, or, in some cases, eliminate the need for penetrating keratoplasty.

Patients not successful with corneal lenses due to poor visual acuity may benefit from a trial with a gas permeable scleral lens. If the poor visual acuity is attributable to an unstable or poorly centered lens, the scleral lens may improve the vision to a functional level. If, however, the reduced visual acuity is due to scarring along the visual axis, a scleral lens will not improve the visual acuity over that provided by a rigid corneal lens. In these cases, penetrating keratoplasty is indicated.

Contact Lens "Troubleshooting"

The skilled contact lens practitioner fitting keratoconus patients spends much of his or her time evaluating contact lens performance in light of patients' signs and symptoms and adjusting contact lens parameters and solutions to change that performance. Sometimes it is as random as "trying something different," but in general, there are tried and true methods for dealing with certain problems.

Inadequate Lens Movement
In keratoconus, it is common that a steep-fitting lens or a lens that appears flat centrally with a too-tight peripheral curve system will not move adequately. Patients with this problem articulate it quite precisely: they describe their lenses as immobile late in the day or with increased hours of wear. The most frequent cause is inadequate edge lift from too-steep peripheral curves. The peripheral curve system can be modified as described below to flatten and blend the secondary and tertiary curves to enhance tear exchange, increase edge lift, and result in a more mobile lens. Occasionally, the central fluorescein pattern of an excessively steep lens must be changed to a flatter fit to achieve the same end.

Poor Visual Acuity
Patients with keratoconus often complain of poor visual acuity with their contact lenses. Often, their complaints outweigh findings on high contrast visual acuity measures in-office. This may be attributable to abnormal contrast sensitivity.[42–45] Anecdotally, practitioners report improved vision with flat-fitting lenses, usually described as the effect of pressure on the apex of the cone resulting in decreased irregular astigmatism. However, this observation has not been duplicated under laboratory conditions.[94]

Nonetheless, keratoconus patients suffer from decreased vision that can often be mitigated by clinical intervention. First and foremost, an accurate overrefraction with the best-fitting rigid contact lenses in place should be performed. In the case of a spherical over-refraction that improves acuity, the power of the contact lenses can be adjusted. If the overrefraction has a significant cylindrical component and the practitioner does not elect to switch to a toric lens design, the spherocylindrical overrefraction can be provided in spectacles to be worn over the contact lenses. Poor vision with steep-fitting lenses may be solved by a switch to flatter-fitting lenses, provided the corneal epithelium can withstand the increased trauma. It is rare that a switch to a piggyback system results in increased visual acuity.

Poor Lens Centration

Keratoconus patients are notorious for decentered lenses. All the usual tricks of the trade can be employed to improve centration: edge design to maximize lid attachment, use of a larger lens to cover the visual axis inside a decentered lens, etc. However, it is the inferior, displaced nature of the cone and the corneal apex that makes changing centration difficult. The lens tends to center over the steepest part of the cornea, which is markedly displaced in this disease. Often, attempts to improve lens centration in a more conventional way result in undesirable changes in lens fit or best-corrected visual acuity.

Rapidly Changing Lens Fit

It often seems as if one or both eyes of a keratoconus patient change from day to day in terms of contact lens fit. Lenses that appear to be functioning well on one visit may be extremely problematic on the next. One rule of thumb is to allow adequate settling time during rigid contact lens fitting visits as described above. If a lens is allowed to settle on a keratoconic cornea for only a few minutes, it is likely that the fit of that lens one week after dispensing may appear very different. This is especially true if a large change is being made in the fitting philosophy, e.g., changing a cornea that has been in a very flat-fitting lens to something considerably steeper. Another rule of thumb is always to dispense a lens unless the visual acuity provided by the lens is completely unacceptable. Lenses that look ill-fitting at a dispensing visit may be quite acceptable at subsequent follow-up visits.

Corneal Staining

Corneal staining is most commonly observed after the instillation of fluorescein onto the inferior or superior bulbar conjunctiva and observation with a slit lamp biomicroscope using either cobalt and yellow filters or white light and moderate magnification and an approximately 2-mm wide slit beam.

The staining should be recorded according to its:

- type (e.g., foreign body, arc, central erosion, swirl, peripheral "3 and 9 o'clock," hypertrophied scar/proud nebula, etc.)

- severity or grade such as:
    0: not observed

    1: minimal, superficial and clinically inconsequential

    2: easily noticeable, requiring monitoring but continued contact lens wear (if contact lens related)

    3: advanced/moderate, coalesced requiring treatment and discontinuation or reduction of contact lens wear

    4: severe, (nearly) maximum, requires rigorous treatment.[107]

Swirl staining may be present prior to contact lens wear in keratoconus and may worsen with contact lens wear. It may be associated with the abnormal enzyme levels in the epithelium and resultant possible aberrant epithelial healing or from the rigid gas permeable lens rotating on the eye. When swirl staining becomes excessive and rigid lens–wearing patients are symptomatic with discomfort and reduced wearing time, then scheduled, heavy-duty cleaning of the back surface of the lens may help. Possibly, an apical clearance, minimal apical touch, or a piggyback contact lens fit may be required. Control of wearing time, with one hour pre- and post-sleep rest from lens wear to allow more normal epithelial healing may also be helpful.

Foreign body staining is characterized by the random appearance of a number of disconnected or overlapping lines. The patient may or may not remember a particle getting under the lens. This staining is typically superficial and does not require treatment. If a contact lens cracks or a large particle causes a foreign body abrasion, lens wear may be discontinued. If symptoms are severe, prophylactic antibiotic, anti-inflammatory, and even bandage contact lens therapy may be administered.

Arc staining in the paracentral cornea may result from a lens that does not move adequately and has a too-sharp junction between the base curve and secondary curve or between other peripheral curves. Heavier blending of the junctions and flattening of the secondary and peripheral curves with added blending are needed to resolve this staining. It is prevented by making sure the base curve and secondary curve junction is not too abrupt to begin with by ordering a secondary curve that is only about 1.00 mm flatter than the base curve with heavy blending. Well-blended third and fourth spherical peripheral curves or aspheric peripheral curves are then needed to obtain adequate edge lift and tear flow. Where normal rigid gas permeable lenses may have about a 0.12 mm axial edge lift, keratoconus lenses may have 0.25 mm axial edge lift.

Proud nebulae or hypertrophied epithelial staining is round and raised and associated with superficial corneal scarring. Although rarely seen in non–contact lens wearers, this condition is best managed by cessation of lens wear if possible, until it heals, and then lens refitting. It can also be surgically removed by hand or with phototherapeutic keratectomy.[51] After healing following surgical removal, rigid gas permeable lens wear is typically much better.

Central corneal epithelial abrasion can be a combined process of the abnormal epithelium in keratoconus, swirl staining, abrasion from the rigid contact lens touching the corneal apex, and deposit formation on the posterior surface of the lens. The first step to resolve this staining—which usually brings the patient to the office with a history of gradual reduction of wearing time and moderate to severe pain—is abstinence from lens wear until the abrasion has been healed for about three to ten days. Once the staining is minimal or, better yet, totally resolved, typically a steeper lens with apical clearance or minimal apical touch will resolve the problem. These lenses are typically 8.5 mm or less in diameter with adequate edge lift and blending. Teaching the patient to clean the lens's posterior surface consistently and control of wearing time are necessary. In some cases, especially with a wide (sagging, oval)[67] cone, the practitioner will have to resort to a large apical-touch fitting lens without excessive inferior edge liftoff. This lens will position consistently with the upper lid. In these cases, back surface cleaning is very important also. In some cases of recurrent central abrasion a piggyback prescription is needed, either on an ongoing basis or as part of the treatment for the recurrent abrasion, especially if spectacle vision or vision with one eye wearing a contact lens is inadequate.

Peripheral corneal ("three and nine o'clock") staining is not as common in keratoconus as it is in normal patients wearing rigid gas permeable lenses. However, minimizing it to protect the limbus and peripheral cornea from neovascularization is important because such vascularization could complicate future penetrating keratoplasty. Whether using a small apical clearance, a three-point touch lens design, or a large lens design, peripheral corneal staining is minimized by assuring: 1) good edge lift, neither too minimal to abrade the peripheral cornea nor too much to cause tear breakup, 2) good edge thickness and shape, 3) consistent blinking, 4) avoiding dry eye by avoiding low humidity and smoky environments, medicines that cause diuresis, and caffeine, and keeping the patient hydrated, 5) lubricants prior to, during, and after lens wear, 6) decrease in wearing time to only work and travel hours, and 7) control of eyelid disease. All of these factors must be applied to assure minimal peripheral staining.

Poor Comfort

Asthenopia in keratoconus is a combination of blur and glare, the typically associated atopic disease, possibly the tendency toward neuroses, and, primarily, the need for a rigid contact lens. Nevertheless, the practitioner must try to keep contact lens wear as optimal as possible. Most lenses that are fitted too flat are uncomfortable at dispensing due to excessive movement and poor lens position (although lenses rarely center on keratoconus corneas), and little improvement in comfort is seen with time. Flat lenses may also have gaps or bubbles under the peripheral lens edge, which can cause epithelial drying and abrasion. Most lenses that are fitted too steep are comfortable initially, but comfort worsens as the lens settles into the malleable keratoconus cornea, trapping debris and possibly bubbles behind the lens.

In advanced keratoconus the lens may have high minus power, thus edge thickness and shape are critical. This requires a lenticular design with an unfinished edge thickness of about 0.12 mm and edge shape with the apex in the middle or posterior one-third of the edge contour.

The reader is directed to the treatment plan for peripheral corneal staining above to prevent lens and ocular drying, which can cause poor comfort.

Lens Modification

The practitioner who does not have modification equipment in the office will have much difficulty with moderate or advanced cases of keratoconus. Most local rigid lens laboratories can help the contact lens practitioner acquire the necessary equipment. The most common equipment and some special modifications are listed below.

Re-edging

Typically, edges from laboratories are too thick rather than too thin. Thinning the edge is most easily done by centering the lens on a lens holder, convex side out, and using water on a diamond cone tool (90 degree) gently so as to uniformly and evenly grind material from the front of the edge. This area is then polished with a tape-covered tool using copious amounts of polish. Then the edge is rounded by spinning a flat sponge into the front of the edge (as it is spun on the sponge) to move the apex back or by spinning the sponge into the back of the edge (as it is spun on the sponge) to move the apex forward (if it is too thin and the apex is too posterior). Copious amounts of polish are used.

Reducing Optic Zone Size (Back Optic Zone Sagittal Depth)

A radius tool (diamond) with a radius of curvature about 1 mm flatter than the base curve is used to evenly and uniformly (using water on the tool) remove about 0.3 mm (wide) of the posterior surface. The area is then polished with copious amounts of polish using a tape- or pad-covered tool of the same radius. Then the lens is blended.

Blending Concentrically or Off Center

Using a tape- or soft pad-covered tool with radius of curvature halfway between the base and secondary curves and copious amounts of polish, the posterior junction is uniformly and evenly blended.

For corneas with a low and not-too-wide cone, an off-center blending (and even flattening the lens more on one side than the other on the posterior surface) can provide a lens that will orient with the flatter posterior area superiorly and the steeper area inferiorly. This is good for cases where adequate peripheral flattening for the flatter superior cornea yields edge standoff inferiorly. This is performed by tilting the lens during peripheral flattening and blending so that one side is blended more than the other.

Increasing Edge Lift

Some laboratories, unless they know that a lens is for a keratoconus patient, may believe that your very flat (relative to the base curve) peripheral curve is incorrect, and the laboratory will make its own version of a standard peripheral curve system. This results in a tight periphery on a lens fitted with apical clearance or minimal apical touch. This can be modified in-office starting with tools with radius of curvature of about 10.0 or 10.5 mm with the lens centered on a lens holder, concave out. The periphery is then uniformly flattened using a diamond tool and polished with a tape- or pad-covered tool using copious amounts of polishing compound.

It is not uncommon to need radii of curvature of 12 to even 17 mm on some keratoconic corneas.

Once the peripheral curve has been adequately flattened, the lens is blended, cleaned, soaked, and applied to the patient. The need for additional modification can then be assessed. Significant peripheral curve flattening may cause a knife edge, and reedging the lens (polishing the posterior edge to move the apex forward) may be necessary, which may decrease the overall lens diameter. This may not be a problem because such higher minus lenses have substantial midperipheral thickness. If modification is not adequate a new lens can be ordered with the knowledge of the necessary design better indicated from the observation of the results of the modifications.

Practicing all of these techniques is recommended prior to applying them to patients' actual lenses. One may choose to have the laboratory perform more specialized (e.g., off-center optic zone) designs. The lens should always be inspected for damage after modification. The modified lens should be cleaned and soaked in a clean case prior to dispensing. All modification tools used, modifications made, and resulting lens diameters should be carefully recorded in the patient's chart.

Indications for Surgery

On average, 10% to 20% of keratoconus patients will need surgery.[4, 6, 7, 71, 108] Surgery is the accepted therapy when contact lenses provide adequate vision but cannot be tolerated, when contact lenses can be tolerated but do not provide adequate acuity, or when the cone extends so far toward the limbus that further progression may make corneal transplantation difficult. Krachmer et al.[1] state that the first two reasons are more common, the third occurring rarely. Keratoplasty for keratoconus is highly successful since the peripheral cornea usually is normal.

Several authors have examined the contact lens and surgical histories of their keratoconus patients to determine what proportion of patients referred for corneal surgery actually are unable to be fitted with contact lenses. Smiddy et al.[71] report that fewer than 13% of 115 consecutive keratoconus patients could not be fitted with contact lenses. Fifty-six percent of prekeratoplasty eyes needed more than three contact lenses over a five-year period. Sixty percent of 88 postoperative eyes needed to wear contact lenses for best vision. Keratoplasty can be delayed or avoided by using contact lenses. This was true in 69% of their selected patients followed for an average of five years[71] and is emphasized by Kastl[78] for 95% of their 64 patients followed for up to 20 years. Belin et al.[109] and Fowler et al.[110] were able to refit 29 of 33 patients originally classified as surgical candidates with 85% achieving visual acuity of at least 20/30. These studies underscore the importance of rigid contact lens correction in keratoconus for patients who never proceed to surgical intervention, in patients thought to be surgical candidates, and in postoperative cases.

It is important that the keratoconus patient be counseled adequately about the unknown etiology of keratoconus, that its course is somewhat unpredictable, and that it does not cause absolute blindness. Even early on, patients are often concerned about the possibility of corneal surgery, and they should know that the chances of that are as low as 1 in 10, that surgery is very successful, and that ongoing care—pre- and/or post-surgically—is the key to managing keratoconus.

Summary

Keratoconus is both a frustrating and a fascinating disease. To treat it, the contact lens practitioner utilizes both the most scientific and the most artistic aspects of his or her profession. Keratoconus can require routine refractive error correction, the most subtle anterior segment disease detection, complicated contact lens correction, and surgical applications within its typical course. This book defines aspects common to the disease; each doctor caring for keratoconus patients can debate the range of its presentation.

References

1. Krachmer JH, Feder RS, Belin MW. Keratoconus and related noninflammatory corneal thinning disorders. Surv Ophthalmol 1984;28:293–322.
2. Duke-Elder S, Leigh AG. Keratoconus. In Systems of Ophthalmology: Diseases of the Outer Eye. Henry Kimpton, 1965;964–976.
3. Hofstetter HW. A keratoscopic survey of 13,395 eyes. Am J Optom Arch Am Acad Optom 1959;36:3–11.
4. Kennedy RH, Bourne WM, Dyer JA. A 48-year clinical and epidemiologic study of keratoconus. Am J Ophthalmol 1986;101:267–273.
5. Amsler M. Le keratocone fruste au javal. Ophthalmol 1938;96:77–83.
6. Eggink FAGJ, Pinckers AJLG, van Puyenbroek EP, et al. Keratoconus, a retrospective study. Cont Lens J 1988;16:204–206.
7. Zadnik K, Gordon MO, Barr JT, et al. Biomicroscopic signs and disease severity in keratoconus. Cornea 1996;15:139–146.
8. Maumenee IH. The cornea in connective tissue disease. Ophthalmol 1978;85:1014–1017.
9. Pierse D, Eustace P. Acute keratoconus in mongols. Br J Ophthalmol 1971;55:50–54.
10. Karel I. Keratoconus in congenital diffuse tapetoretinal degeneration. Ophthalmologica 1968;155:8–15.
11. Copeman PW. Eczema and keratoconus. Br Med J 1965;2:977–979.
12. Gasset AR, Hinson WA, Frias JL. Keratoconus and atopic diseases. Ann Ophthalmol 1978;10:991–994.
13. Khan MD, Kundi N, Saud N, et al. Incidence of keratoconus in sping catarrh. Br J Ophthalmol 1988;72:41–43.
14. Rahi A, Davies P, Ruben M, et al. Keratoconus and coexisting atopic disease. Br J Ophthalmol 1977;61:761–764.
15. Gasset AR, Houde WL, Garcia-Bengochea M. Hard contact lens wear as an environmental risk in keratoconus. Am J Ophthalmol 1978;85:339–341.
16. Hartstein J. Corneal warping. Am J Ophthalmol 1965;60:1103–1104.
17. Hartstein J. Keratoconus that developed in patients wearing corneal contact lenses. Arch Ophthalmol 1968;80:728–729.
18. Hartstein J. Keratoconus and contact lenses. J Am Med Assoc 1969;208:539.
19. Gritz DC, McDonnell PJ. Keratoconus and ocular massage. Am J Ophthalmol 1988;106:757–758.
20. Karseras AG, Ruben M. Aetiology of keratoconus. Br J Ophthalmol 1976;60:522–525.
21. Ridley F. Eye-rubbing and contact lenses. Br J Ophthalmol 1961;45:631.

22. Hartstein J, Becker B. Research into the pathogenesis of keratoconus: a new syndrome: Low ocular rigidity, contact lenses, and keratoconus. Arch Ophthalmol 1970;84:728–729.
23. Davies PD, Ruben M. The paretic pupil: its incidence and etiology after keratoplasty for keratoconus. Br J Ophthalmol 1975;59:223–228.
24. Brooks AMV, Robertson IF, Mahoney A-M. Ocular rigidity and intraocular pressure in keratoconus. Aust J Ophthalmol 1984;12:317–324.
25. Foster CS, Yamamoto GK. Ocular rigidity in keratoconus. Am J Ophthalmol 1978;86:802–806.
26. Andreassen TT., Simonsen AH., Oxlund, H. Biomechanical properties of keratoconus and normal corneas. Exp Eye Res 1980;31:435–441.
27. Newsome DA, Foidart JM, Hassell JR, et al. Detection of specific collagen types in normal and keratoconus corneas. Invest Ophthalmol Vis Sci 1981;20:738–750.
28. Rehany U, Lahav M, Shoshan S. Collagenolytic activity in keratoconus. Ann Ophthalmol 1982;14:751–754.
29. Yue BYJT, Panjwani N, Sugar J, et al. Glycoconjugate abnormalities in cultured keratoconus stromal cells. Arch Ophthalmol 1988;106:1709–1712.
30. Yue BYJT, Sugar J, Benveniste K. Heterogeneity in keratoconus: possible biochemical basis. Proc Soc Exp Biol Med 1984;175:336–341.
31. Yue BYJT, Sugar J, Schrode K. Histochemical studies in keratoconus. Curr Eye Res 1988;7:81–86.
32. Fukuchi T, Yue BYJT, Sugar J, et al. Lysosomal enzyme activities in conjunctival tissues of patients with keratoconus. Arch Ophthalmol 1994;112:1368–1374.
33. Sawaguchi S, Twining SS, Yue BYJT, et al. a2-macroglobulin levels in normal human and keratoconus corneas. Invest Ophthalmol Vis Sci 1994;35:4008–4014.
34. Sawaguchi S, Twining SS, Yue BYJT, et al. a1-proteinase inhibitor levels in keratoconus. Exp Eye Res 1990;50:549–554.
35. Zadnik K, Barr JT, Edrington TB, Everett DF, Jameson M, McMakon TT, Sterling JL, Wagner H, Gordon MD, and the CLEK Study Group. Baseline findings in the Collaborative Longitudinal Evaluation of Keratoconus (CLEK) Study. Invest Ophthalmol Vis Sci (in press).
36. Lowell FS, Carroll JM. A study of the occurrence of atopic traits in patients with keratoconus. J All Clin Immunol 1970;46:32–39.
37. Wachtmeister L, Ingemansson S, Moller E. Atopy and HLA antigens in patents with keratoconus. Acta Ophthalmol 1982;60:113–122.
38. Zadnik K, Mannis MJ, Johnson CA. An analysis of contrast sensitivity in identical twins with keratoconus. Cornea 1984;3:99–103.

39. Hammerstein W. Zur genetik des keratoconus. Albrecht von Graefes Arch Klin Exp Ophthalmol 1974;190:293–308.

40. Rabinowitz YS, Garbus J, McDonnell PJ. Computer-assisted corneal topography in family members of patients with keratoconus. Arch Ophthalmol 1990;108:365–371.

41. Gordon MO, Schechtman KB, Davis LJ, et al. Repeatability of visual acuity in keratoconus: impact on sample size. Optom Vis Sci 1998;75:249–257.

42. Carney LG. Contact lens correction of visual loss in keratoconus. Acta Ophthalmol 1982;60:795–802.

43. Carney LG. Visual loss in keratoconus. Arch Ophthalmol 1982;100:1282–1285.

44. Mannis MJ, Zadnik K, Johnson CA, et al. Contrast sensitivity after penetrating keratoplasty. Arch Ophthalmol 1987;105:1220–1223.

45. Zadnik K, Mannis MJ, Johnson CA, et al. Rapid contrast sensitivity assessment in keratoconus. Am J Optom Physiol Opt 1987;64:693–697.

46. Swann PG, Waldron HE. Keratoconus: the clinical spectrum. J Am Optom Assoc 1986;57:204–209.

47. Edmund C. Assessment of an elastic model in the pathogenesis of keratoconus. Acta Ophthalmol 1987;65:545–550.

48. Vogt A. Reflexlinien durch faltung spiegelnder grenzflachen im bereiche von corneo, linsenkapsel und netzhaut. Albrecht von Graefes Arch Ophthalmol 1919;99:296–338.

49. Fanta H. Acute keratoconus. In JG Bellows (ed), Contemporary Ophthalmology. Baltimore, MD Williams & Wilkins, 1972;64–68.

50. Korb DR, Finnemore VM, Herman JP. Apical changes and scarring in keratoconus as related to contact lens fitting techniques. J Am Optom Assoc 1982;53:199–205.

51. Moodaley L, Buckley RJ, Woodward EG. Surgery to improve contact lens wear in keratoconus. CLAO J 1991;17:129–131.

52. Barr JT, Gordon MO, Zadnik K, et al. Photodocumentation of corneal scarring. J Refr Surg 1996;12:492–500.

53. Mandell RB, Polse KA. Keratoconus: spatial variation of corneal thickness as a diagnostic tool. Arch Ophthalmol 1969;82:182–188.

54. Gromacki SJ, Barr JT. Central and peripheral corneal thickness in keratoconus and normal patient groups. Optom Vis Sci 1994;71:437–441.

55. Poster MG, Gelfer DM, Greenwald I, et al. An optical classification of keratoconus—a preliminary report. Am J Optom Arch Am Acad Optom 1968;45:216–230.

56. Shaw EL, Sewell J, Gasset AR. Photodiagnosis of keratoconus. Ann Ophthalmol 1973;3:297–300.

57. Rizzuti AB. Diagnostic illumination test for keratoconus. Am J Ophthalmol 1970;70:141–143.

58. Appelbaum A. Keratoconus. Arch Ophthalmol 1936;15:900–921.
59. Maguire LJ, Bourne WM. Corneal topography of early keratoconus. Am J Ophthalmol 1989;108:107–112.
60. Maguire LJ, Lowry JC. Identifying progression of subclinical keratoconus by serial topography analysis. Am J Ophthalmol 1991;112:41–45.
61. McMahon TT, Robin JB, Scarpulla KM, et al. The spectrum of topography found in keratoconus. CLAO J 1991;17:198–204.
62. Rabinowitz YS, McDonnell PJ. Computer-assisted corneal topography in keratoconus. Refr Corn Surg 1989;5:400–408.
63. Nesburn AB, Bahri S, Salz J, et al. Keratoconus detected by videokeratography in candidates for photorefractive keratectomy. J Refr Surg 1995;11:194–201.
64. Hannush SB, Crawford SL, Waring GO, et al. Accuracy and precision of keratometry, photokeratoscopy, and corneal modeling on calibrated steel balls. Arch Ophthalmol 1989;107:1235–1239.
65. Hannush SB, Crawford SL, Waring GO, et al. Reproducibility of normal corneal power measurements with a keratometer, photokeratoscope, and video imaging system. Arch Ophthalmol 1990;108:539–544.
66. Heath GG, Gerstman DR, Wheeler WH, et al. Reliability and validity of videokeratoscopic measurements. Optom Vis Sci 1991;68:946–949.
67. Caroline PJ, McGuire JR, Doughman DJ. Preliminary report on a new contact lens design for keratoconus. Cont Int Lens Med J 1978;4:69–73.
68. Perry HD, Buxton JN, Fine BS. Round and oval cones in keratoconus. Ophthalmol 1980;87:905–909.
69. Besançon G, Baikoff G, Deneux A, et al. Note preliminaire sur l'etat psychologique et mental des porteurs de keratocone. Bull Soc Ophthalmol Fr. 1980;80:4–5.
70. Mannis MJ, Morrison TL, Zadnik K, et al. Personality trends in keratoconus: an analysis. Arch Ophthalmol 1987;105:798–800.
71. Smiddy WE, Hamburg TR, Kracher GP, et al. Keratoconus: contact lens or keratoplasty? Ophthalmol 1988;95:487–492.
72. Davis LJ, Schechtman KB, Begley CG, et al. Repeatability of refraction and corrected visual acuity in keratoconus. Optom Vis Sci (in press).
73. Lowther GE. Optics of contact lenses. In N Bier, GE Lowther (eds), Contact Lens Correction. Boston: Butterworths, 1977;34.
74. Cohen EJ, Parlato CJ. Fitting Polycon lenses in keratoconus. Int Ophthalmol Clin 1986;26:111–117.
75. Gasset AR, Lobo L. Dura-T semiflexible lenses for keratoconus. Ann Ophthalmol 1975;7:1353–1357.
76. Gould HE. Management of keratoconus with corneal and scleral lenses. Am J Ophthalmol 1970;70:624–629.

77. Hall KGC. A comprehensive study of keratoconus. Br J Physiol Opt 1963;20:215–256.

78. Kastl PR. A 20-year retrospective study of the use of contact lenses in keratoconus. CLAO J 1987;13:102–104.

79. Lembach RG, Keates RH. Aspheric silicone lenses for keratoconus. CLAO J 1984;10:323–325.

80. Mackie I. Management of keratoconus with hard corneal lenses: the lens lid attachment technique. Trans Ophthalmol Soc UK 1977;97:131–135.

81. Maguen E, Espinosa G, Rosner IR, et al. Long-term wear of Polycon contact lenses in keratoconus. CLAO J 1983;9:57–59.

82. Mobilia EF, Foster CS. A one-year trial of Polycon lenses in the correction of keratoconus. Cont Int Lens Med J 1979;5:37–42.

83. Raber IM. Use of CAB Soper Cone contact lenses in keratoconus. CLAO J 1983;9:237–240.

84. Rosenthal P. The Boston lens and the management of keratoconus. Int Ophthalmol Clin 1986;26:101–109.

85. Soper JW, Jarrett A. Results of a systematic approach to fitting keratoconus and corneal transplants. Cont Lens Med Bull 1972;5:50–59.

86. Voss EH, Liberatore JC. Fitting the apex of keratoconus. Contacto 1962;6:212–214.

87. Brady HR. Keratoconus development in a contact lens wearer. Cont Lens Med Bull 1972;5:23.

88. Brightbill FS, Stainer GA. Previous hard contact lens wear in keratoconus. Cont Int Lens Med J 1979;5:43–47.

89. Steahly LP. Keratoconus following contact lens wear. Ann Ophthalmol 1978;10:1177–1179.

90. Ederer F, Ferris FL. Studying the role of an environmental factor in disease etiology (letter to the editor). Am J Ophthalmol 1979;86:434–435.

91. Sommer A. Keratoconus in contact lens wear (letter to the editor). Am J Ophthalmol 1978;86:442–444.

92. Macsai MS, Varley GA, Krachmer JH. Development of keratoconus after contact lens wear. Arch Ophthalmol 1990;108:435–538.

93. Krachmer JH. Pellucid marginal corneal degeneration. Arch Ophthalmol 1978;96:1217–1221.

94. Zadnik K, Mutti DO. Contact lens fitting relation and visual acuity in keratoconus. Am J Optom Physiol Opt 1987;64:698–702.

95. Mandell RB. Keratoconus. In RB Mandell (ed), Contact Lens Practice. Springfield, IL: Charles C Thomas, 1988;732–751.

96. Bennett ES. Keratoconus. In ES Bennett and RM Grohe (eds), Rigid Gas Permeable Contact Lenses. Chapel Hill, NC: Professional Press Books, 1986; pp. 297–394.

97. Edrington TB, Barr JT, Zadnik K, et al. Standardized rigid contact lens fitting protocol for keratoconus. Optom Vis Sci 1996;73:369–375.

98. Edrington TB, Szczotka LB, Begley CG, et al. Repeatability and agreement of two corneal curvature assessments in keratoconus: keratometry and the first definite apical clearance lens (FDACL). Cornea 1998;17:267–277.

99. Koliopoulos J, Tragakis M. Visual correction of keratoconus with soft contact lenses. Ann Ophthalmol 1981;13:835–837.

100. Tragakis MP, Brown SI. Hydrophilic lenses for correcting irregular and high astigmatism. Arch Ophthalmol 1972;88:596–601.

101. Baldone JA. The fitting of hard contact lenses onto soft contact lenses in certain diseased conditions. Cont Lens Med Bull 1973;6:15–17.

102. Zadnik K, Mannis MJ. The use of the Saturn II lens in keratoconus and corneal transplant patients. Int Cont Lens Clin 1987;14:312–315.

103. Pullum KW, Hobley AJ, Davison C. 110+ Dk: does thickness make much difference? J Br Cont Lens Assoc 1991;6:158–161.

104. Ezekiel D. Gas permeable haptic lenses. J Br Cont Lens Assoc 1983;6:158–161.

105. Schein OD, Rosenthal P, Ducharme C. A gas permeable scleral contact lens for visual rehabilitation. Am J Ophthalmol 1990;109:318–322.

106. Pullum KW. Feasibility study for the production of gas permeable scleral lenses using ocular impression techniques. Trans Br Cont Lens Assoc 1987;10:35–39.

107. Barr JT. The Cornea. In K Zadnik (ed), The Ocular Examination Measurements and Findings. Philadelphia: Saunders, 1996;211.

108. Sayegh FN, Ehlers N, Farah I. Evaluation of penetrating keratoplasty in keratoconus: nine years follow-up. Acta Ophthalmol 1988;66:400–403.

109. Belin MW, Fowler WG, and Chambers WA. Keratoconus: evaluation of recent trends in the surgical and nonsurgical correction of keratoconus. Ophthalmol. 1988;95:335–337.

110. Fowler WC, Belin MW, Chambers WA. Contact lenses in the visual correction of keratoconus. CLAO J 1988;14:203–206.

Index

Notes

Notes

Notes

Notes

Notes